POCKET GUIDES

CW00924632

PHYSICIAN ASSOCIATE PLACEMENTS

POCKET GUIDES

A unique series of pocket-sized books designed to help healthcare students make the most of their practice learning experiences.

"All the information was clear and concise, this book is exactly what I was looking for." ★★★★★

"A great little guide. All the basic information needed to have a quick reference." ★★★★★

"A very useful, well-written and practical pocket book for any level of student nurse preparing for placement." ★★★★★

"Written by students for students. A must for any student about to head on placement." ★★★★★

POCKET GUIDES

PHYSICIAN ASSOCIATE PLACEMENTS

Kate Straughton
University of Birmingham

Jeannie Watkins
St George's, University of London

Lantern

ISBN 9781908625984
First published in 2022 by Lantern Publishing Ltd

Lantern Publishing Limited, The Old Hayloft, Vantage
Business Park, Bloxham Road, Banbury OX16 9UX, UK
www.lanternpublishing.com

British Library Cataloguing in Publication Data
A catalogue record for this book is available from the British Library

The authors and publisher have made every attempt to ensure
the content of this book is up to date and accurate. However,
healthcare knowledge and information is changing all the time
so the reader is advised to double-check any information in
this text on drug usage, treatment procedures, the use of
equipment, etc. to confirm that it complies with the latest safety
recommendations, standards of practice and legislation, as well as
local Trust policies and procedures. Students are advised to check
with their tutor and/or practice supervisor before carrying out
any of the procedures in this textbook.

Typeset by Medlar Publishing Solutions Pvt Ltd, India
Printed and bound in the UK

Last digit is the print number: 10 9 8 7 6 5 4

Personal information

Name:. . . . .

Mobile:. . . . .

Address during placement:. . . . .

UNIVERSITY DETAILS

University: . . . .

Programme leader: . . . .

Personal tutor:. . . . .

PLACEMENT DETAILS

Placement area:. . . . .

Practice Education Facilitator:. . . . .

Link lecturer: . . . .

CONTACT IN CASE OF EMERGENCY

Name:. . . . .

Contact number (mobile): . . . .

Contact number (home/work): . . . .

Contents

Moving on

Resources

Preface

We believe that PA students are strong, visible ambassadors who can help the NHS understand what a PA can do, and how PAs fit into the team. Hopefully, for PA students just starting your journey, this book will get you thinking about the importance of clinical placements, how vital it is to be prepared for placement, to participate when you are there, to optimise your time and learning opportunities (knowing what you can contribute and what you can get from the placement). This book should also enable you to reflect and learn from your experiences. We also hope that his handbook will make the clinical placement experience a little less scary and enable you to prepare for working life as a newly qualified PA.

Kate Straughton

Jeannie Watkins

Acknowledgements

Having worked as Physician Associates in roles (clinical and academic) supporting PA students on their clinical placements for many years, we would like to extend a huge thank you to all the students we have worked with. Without you, your questions, concerns, ideas, challenges, and oodles of examples of brilliant practice, we would not have anything to say!

Thank you also to those colleagues (Tripti Chakraborty, Kay Ling, Wendi Heathcock, Ruth Berry and Dr Iram Khattak) and PA students (Gabriella Smith, Louis Menson Evans, Ealish Brew and Balraj Pandher) who have reviewed this book. Your constructive feedback – comments and suggestions based on your wide and varied experiences of clinical placements – was thoughtful, pragmatic and incredibly helpful. We are grateful for your contributions. Also, our thanks to the General Medical Council for permission to use the professional standards for medical healthcare professionals and students and apply those to PAs.

Abbreviations

Below you will find abbreviations used in this book. There is also space for you to create a list of further (approved) abbreviations that you encounter during placement.

Familiarise yourself with locally approved abbreviations in your first few days of placement.

A&E	Accident and Emergency
ABC	Airway, breathing, circulation
ABG	Arterial blood gas
ACE	Angiotensin-converting enzyme
ACVPU	Alert, new Confusion, responds to Voice, responds to Pain, Unresponsive
ADLs	Activities of daily living
AHP	Allied Health Professional
ALs	Activities of living
ARDS	Acute respiratory distress syndrome
BLS	Basic life support
BP	Blood pressure
C. diff	*Clostridium difficile*
CA	Cancer
CD	Controlled drug
CHF	Chronic heart failure
COPD	Chronic obstructive pulmonary disease
CPD	Continuing professional development
CPR	Cardiopulmonary resuscitation
CSU	Catheter specimen urine
CVA	Cerebrovascular accident (stroke)
DNAR	Do not attempt resuscitation
DOB	Date of birth
DOPS	Direct Observation of Procedural Skills

DVT	Deep vein thrombosis
ECG	Electrocardiogram
ED	Emergency department
ENT	Ear, nose and throat
ET	Endotracheal tube
GCS	Glasgow Coma Scale
GMC	General Medical Council
H_2O	Water
HIV	Human immunodeficiency virus
HR	Heart rate
HTN	Hypertension
I&D	Incision and drainage
I&O	Intake and output
IBS	Irritable bowel syndrome
ICP	Intracranial pressure
ICU/ITU	Intensive care unit / intensive treatment unit
IM	Intramuscular
INH	Inhaled
IV	Intravenous
LOC	Level / loss of consciousness
MDT	Multidisciplinary team
MRSA	Methicillin-resistant *Staphylococcus aureus*
MSU	Midstream urine specimen
NBM	Nil by mouth
NG	Nasogastric
NSAID	Non-steroidal anti-inflammatory drug
O	Oral
O_2	Oxygen

PE	Pulmonary embolism
PGD	Patient Group Direction
PPE	Personal protective equipment
PR	Per rectum
PRN	As needed
PV	Per vagina
RBC	Red blood cell
SBARD	Situation, background, assessment, recommendation, decision
S/C	Subcutaneous
S/L	Sublingual
SOB	Shortness of breath
SPA	Suprapubic aspirate
TIA	Transient ischaemic attack
TOP	Topical *or* Termination of pregnancy
TPN	Total parenteral nutrition
TPR	Temperature, pulse, respiration
UA	Urinalysis
UTI	Urinary tract infection
VRE	Vancomycin-resistant *Enterococcus*
WBC	White blood cell

✎ Note your own (approved) abbreviations

Introduction

Physician Associate programmes are designed to deliver medical knowledge and skills over a minimum of 90 weeks, preparing students for entry into professional practice. At least half of the programme is based in the clinical environment, rotating through a range of core and elective medical and surgical specialties across primary and secondary care. PA student clinical placements are a fundamental part of the educative process, incorporating theory with practice and building confidence and competence. However, it is recognised that placements can also be challenging mentally, physically and financially, and a source of anxiety and stress.

This handbook is a practical guide to help PA students prepare for clinical placements, giving factual and useful information to enable students to function safely, maximise the opportunities available and get the most out of their attachments. It provides general guidance and principles (not specific to any one placement area) applicable to most areas of practice. With good preparation, communication and commitment students stand the best chance of being successful in achieving their objectives and find that placements can be incredibly enriching and rewarding experiences.

Notes

Getting there

Preparing for placement

Preparation for placement is one of the main keys to a successful placement experience. 'Fail to prepare, prepare to fail'. Using the who, when, what, where and how questions is an effective way to start your preparation.

- **Who** will I be working alongside on placement? **Who** will be supervising me? **Who** do I ask if I have any questions or challenges? **Who** will I meet on the first day?
- **When** do I start my placement? **When** do I need to be there? **When** do I finish my placement? **When** do I need to seek help?
- **What** am I going to do on placement? **What** is expected of me? **What** time do I start? **What** time do I finish? **What** do I need to bring with me?
- **Where** is my placement? **Where** do I park? **Where** can I get food and drinks on site? **Where** can I keep my things?
- **How** do I get there? **How** do I get the most out of this specific placement? **How** do I juggle focusing on my learning with patient care? **How** do I prepare to get ID cards/access to the department?

For students with statement of support needs, reasonable adjustments or additional needs, it is good to check that your placement sites are aware of this. This would normally be requested by your university course team, so it is worth confirming with them if they have advised the placement of your needs and if not, that they do. It is also worth mentioning any adjustments that you need in the email to your placement when introducing yourself and seeking first day instructions. This information will help placements prepare for your arrival and enable you to get the most out of your placement.

- Discuss with the placement team on your course – should you be contacting the supervisor ahead of your placement to introduce yourself and find out your reporting instructions? Should you be expecting an email from the supervisor (or colleague) or is it all done on day one?
- Look at the organisation website. Do your homework as you would for a job interview. Consider questions such as:
  - Who runs the organisation? Chief executive, medical director, director of nursing, etc.
  - Who are the undergraduate and postgraduate administrators?
  - What services does it offer? Are these all on one site?
  - What are the different departments in the organisation?
  - Who are the different health professionals employed there?
  - Are there any PAs employed there?
  - Is there an education centre?
- Think about the type of placement that you are going to and what would be relevant to know about that specific placement/specialty.

The answers to these questions will have an impact on the way that your placements function, and how you achieve your placement objectives or clinical skills.

 Notes

As a student you will attend placement as arranged and agreed by your university and the placement provider. Regular, timely attendance is key to ensuring that you can access all the opportunities and experiences available to you, meet placement attendance requirements and demonstrate that as a student you are a consistent, dependable, reliable and visible member of the team.

If you need to attend at a different time to that arranged, then you will need to negotiate this with your PA course team and placement. This is to ensure that the placement has capacity to accommodate you and that there is appropriate supervision in place to support and oversee your learning.

There may be requirements or optional opportunities for flexibility within placement working patterns – for example, in some areas it may be possible to be on placement for four longer days rather than the traditional working week. There will also be the opportunity to experience evenings, nights and weekends in some placements – these should be encouraged but ensure that you have a safe supportive network of qualified colleagues to supervise you, as there are significantly fewer staff around at night. This flexibility might not be available in every area; discuss with your placement team and your supervisors where appropriate.

If you are going to be late or absent from placement, make sure you have the contact details of those you need to inform (placement and university) and let them know as soon as possible about your delay or absence. Effective communication is essential when on placement and is a good demonstration of your professionalism. If you are absent from placement you will need to communicate with the university and placement regarding the reason for the absence and when you will return. Depending on the reason for the absence other people may also need to be made aware; Occupational Health (university and placement site) and your GP. Your course team and the university will advise on this where appropriate.

University absence contact:	
Name/department	
Phone number(s)	
Email	

Placement 1 absence contact:	
Name/department	
Phone number(s)	
Email	

Placement 2 absence contact:	
Name/department	
Phone number(s)	
Email	

Placement 3 absence contact:	
Name/department	
Phone number(s)	
Email	

Placement 4 absence contact:

Name / department	
Phone number(s)	
Email	

Placement 5 absence contact:

Name / department	
Phone number(s)	
Email	

Placement 6 absence contact:

Name / department	
Phone number(s)	
Email	

Placement 7 absence contact:

Name / department	
Phone number(s)	
Email	

Placement 8 absence contact:

Name / department	
Phone number(s)	
Email	

Make sure that you are clear about the learning objectives for each placement and what is required of you. You should also ensure that you relay these to your team/supervisor on your first day. This is particularly helpful when they have not had much experience of working with PA students. If your objectives are not clear or you have no learning objectives, speak to your PA course team. Review the Matrix of Common and Important Conditions[1], using this as a revision guide to identify knowledge or clinical experience gaps. Check which clinical examinations and procedures you need to undertake, and which placement is best suited to carry these out. Confirm the hours or days that you are scheduled to attend, ensuring that you meet the requirements for the programme, getting appropriate sign-off as required. It is best practice to get any time sheets or sign-offs for placement attendance or clinical procedures as you go through the placement. Medical staff rotate and you might find yourself chasing people for sign-offs who have moved on. Bring your placement paperwork with you.

✎ Notes

_____

_____

_____

_____

[1]Note: The FPA/RCP are developing a new curriculum for PA education which will be approved by the GMC following statutory regulation. Once the new curriculum is in place, PA programmes will be required to use this as a structure; the CCF and Matrix will no longer be used.

Challenge yourself – Documentation

Make a list or spreadsheet of all of your placement requirements for each individual placement, and then tick them off as you achieve them. These might include (but are not limited to):

- Direct Observation of Procedural Skills (DOPS) forms
- Multi-source feedback (MSF)
- Case-based discussions
- Placement assessment documents
- Timesheets

Notes

Some useful preparation before you start placements may include tasks such as:

- reading around the common and important conditions, presentations, diagnosis and management and the 'red flags' for each placement
- practising case history and clinical examinations skills to gain more confidence
- speaking to other students who may have been to that placement or on a similar placement at that clinical site.

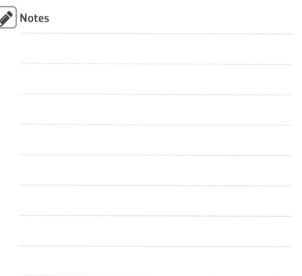 **Notes**

6 Pre-placement modules (organisation-specific)

Some organisations may require students to complete induction modules prior to attending placement. These may be in relation to health and safety, IT training or other training specific to the organisation. You will need to factor in time to complete these, as they can be lengthy. Most organisations will advise students and the university if these need to be completed.

 Notes

Budgeting for placement is essential. Travel costs, parking, eating and drinking can make a huge dent in your finances. There are differences across the UK in terms of funding; discuss with your course team to find out what is available from your course. Flexibility in work patterns (where available) may provide some support by reducing travel costs; however, you should also think about the most cost-effective way of getting to placement; for example, car share, cycling, walking, staying with a friend or relative local to the placement if possible. Consider taking a packed lunch, and bring your own water bottle, flask or reusable cup. Coffee shops at placement sites, while very convenient and offering delicious food and drink, are also expensive. There may be some discount apps, money back apps or student discounts for coffee shops. Hospital canteens are normally a little cheaper and some may also offer student discount.

> You may need ID to access these discounts.

 Notes

It is important that you sort out your route and your mode of transport to placement. It is good to trial your route prior to attending and to do this at the time you would normally be travelling. This will help you with timings and potentially working out alternative routes should they be required. This preparation will help you get to placement on time.

If you drive, you should explore if there is parking, and if so, whether payment is required. If you are expected to pay for car parking, ask if there is a reduced rate for students. It may take a couple of weeks to allocate a permit, so explore this option as far in advance as possible. It is also worth checking out if there is hospital transport (should you need to go between sites) or cycle racks if you decide to travel by bicycle. If you work a later shift, you should check that you will still be able to get home safely with your chosen mode of transport.

1 Top tips – transport

- If you use transport, ensure that you start out extra early on your first day to make sure that you are not late if you run into unanticipated issues. If you do find that you arrive early, it gives you more time to familiarise yourself with the environment and people, or to do some studying!
- Remember to look at the local transport websites to check for the best deals on public transport, e.g. weekly passes or top-up cards.
- Consider carrying out a 'dry run' before starting your placement. If going by car, how long does it take to get from the car park to the building? Where else might you need to park? If going by public transport, consider transfer time, if necessary, as well as then walking to the placement building.

Some placements (mostly acute hospital sites) have accommodation available for students. You may wish to consider contacting your placement to see if this is available; however, you may need to pay for this. As mentioned in *Section 7*, if you have a placement which is a few hours' commute from your home address, then staying with a friend or relative more locally could be helpful, if that is a possibility.

Notes

Equipment

You need to be prepared for placement. Most organisations will have some equipment for students and other clinicians to use; however, there are some items that you may find useful to have. Increasingly, departments are going paperless with electronic records, so check with your Trust as they may prefer you to take your notes on a tablet or other device if you have one available. Be mindful of where you might store valuables and expensive equipment, and make sure your name is clearly identifiable on the equipment.

- Stethoscope
- Pocket ophthalmoscope / otoscope
- Saturation monitor
- Small measuring tape
- Small pocket handbook / textbook
- Pocket notebook and pens / tablet (but be mindful of storage of valuables).

> Remember to bring this book with you!

 Notes

It is important that you dress in a professional manner when on placement (no jeans, T-shirts or trainers). Make sure you have clothes that are both functional and comfortable to wear and that you can move around in easily. Trousers and skirts with pockets are a practical solution, or you may wish to carry a small cross-body bag to keep some key items in. Your PA course, or the placement organisation, may have a dress/uniform policy and it is worth asking about this prior to attending placement. Some placements may expect you to wear scrubs. If they do, make sure to ask somebody where you can get scrubs, if you need instructions such as how to use a scrub machine, and where you can deposit them at the end of the day, as this may be in a different place to where you got them from.

✏ Notes

_____

_____

_____

_____

_____

_____

_____

_____

_____

.2 | Placement schedule

For each placement you should be provided with a placement
schedule from the placement provider. You may be given this
prior to the placement starting or once you start. If you do
not receive one, then it is good to ask about this – you may
have a flexible schedule.

See *Section 26:
Timetable*

 Notes

Whilst on placement it is likely that you will meet and be on the same attachments as other healthcare students. It is good to speak and collaborate with them as part of your learning experience. These students will be your future colleagues. They may wish to know more about your role as PA, and it may be worthwhile exploring their role and how it forms part of the team. You may also wish to share good learning experiences on that placement that are useful for you.

✎ Notes

.4   Placement contacts

Prior to your placements you should be informed of who the contacts are at that organisation and their designations. You should know who your placement supervisor is and have the appropriate contact details for them – keep a record on *page v* of this book. When on placement it is good to confirm who is best to contact in the event of lateness or absence and to have their contact details. You should share only your university email address with those on placement, rather than personal email addresses.

> Use the space at the end of *Section 3* to keep a note of these contact details

 Notes

_____

_____

_____

_____

_____

_____

Prior to attending your placement, the organisation and placement supervisor will be notified in advance of the dates of your placement and any other information required. It is your responsibility to make contact prior to starting your placement to introduce yourself and check for your first day instructions* (where to go and who to report to and what to bring along). If you struggle to contact your placement or do not hear back from them then you should let your PA programme team know in a timely manner. The process of contacting placements and receipt of first day instructions may vary from university to university, but the bottom line is that you should know where you are going and where to show up on the first day and who will be supervising you.

*(Note: only make contact when you have been advised to do so by your course team.)

 Top tip – supervisor meetings

Arrange to meet with your supervisor on your first day to discuss objectives for the placement, what you need to achieve and how you can do this in placement. For longer placements, arrange a meeting midway through to discuss your progression. You should arrange a meeting for the end of your placement to review your performance, gain advice about how to improve moving forward and to get any paperwork signed off. See the table in *Section 34* for more detail.

16 | Smart cards / IT access

As a student you will need to have access to the IT systems in order to be able to participate more fully as part of the team. Your programme team should be able to arrange access with the placement providers. It is likely that the access you may have will be read-only; however, this should be enough for you to be able to participate and engage. Most students will have a smart card to access the systems. If you lose your smart card or are struggling with IT access, then you must let your university and your placement know. Of note, you may be required to undertake additional training to use the IT systems in the organisation.

 Notes

As a PA student on placement, you will be expected to exhibit the professional behaviours and attitudes of a medical healthcare professional. These are defined by the General Medical Council and detailed in *Good Medical Practice: interim standards for physician associates and anaesthesia associates* (2021). In addition to this the GMC has also published guidance for medical students, *Achieving Good Medical Practice* (2016) which explains the standards of professional behaviour as a student. Whilst the latter publication is specifically for medical students, this guidance is relevant to PA students pending regulation with the GMC. We have outlined the main points below, but you should familiarise yourself with both documents. In addition to this your university may also have professionalism expectations that you are required to uphold and demonstrate whilst on placement; again you should be aware of these. The Faculty of Physician Associates has a published Code of Conduct and Scope of Professional Practice for qualified PAs which is based on GMC guidance.

Standards expected for doctors and medical students; also applicable to PAs

Domain 1: Knowledge, skills and performance

Develop and maintain your professional performance

- As a registered PA, you will be expected to keep your skills and knowledge up to date so you can give your patients the best standard of care

Apply knowledge and experience to practice

- PAs must recognise and work within the limits of their competence

Record your work clearly, accurately, and legibly

Domain 2: Safety and quality

- Contribute to and comply with systems to protect patients
- Respond to risks to safety
- Protect patients and colleagues from any risk posed by your health

Domain 3: Communication, partnership and teamwork

- Communicate effectively
- Work collaboratively with colleagues to maintain or improve patient care
- Ensure continuity and coordination of care
- Establish and maintain partnerships with patients
- Maintain patient confidentiality

Domain 4: Maintaining trust

- Show respect for patients
- Treat patients and colleagues fairly and without discrimination
- Act with honesty and integrity

Source: *Good Medical Practice* (GMC, 2021) and *Achieving Good Medical Practice* (GMC, 2016).

 Challenge yourself – Professionalism guidance

Familiarise yourself with the supporting documentation for clinical placements. This includes:

- GMC *Good Medical Practice: interim standards for physician associates and anaesthesia associates*
- GMC *Achieving Good Medical Practice*
- University documentation including handbooks, assessment guidance and professionalism expectations
- Faculty of Physician Associates – Code of Conduct and Scope of Professional Practice.

17.1 Being professional on placements – practical steps

The following steps are taken from the GMC publication *Achieving Good Medical Practice* (2016):

- Always introduce yourself to patients, letting them know your name and that you are a Physician Associate student.
- When you meet a patient for the first time, check if they have any objections to having a student present.
- If your university or placement provider has given you an ID badge or similar, make sure it is always visible.
- Dress smartly and in line with dress codes set out by your university or placement provider.
- Arrive on time for your placement and do not leave your placement early unless you have agreed this with a relevant supervisor.
- Attend induction sessions if they are offered.
- Attend all mandatory training arranged for you while on a placement.
- Make sure you know about and follow the rules and guidance specific to your placement, including how you should raise any concerns. If in doubt, make sure you ask if there is anything in particular you should know at the start of your placement.
- Be honest with patients if you do not know the answer to their questions. Patients appreciate that you are there to learn.
- Make sure you know who is responsible for directly supervising you on your placement and who has the overall responsibility for PA students where you are working. This will help you understand where to go if you need help and if you have any concerns you need to raise.
- Be aware that while on any elective, in the UK or abroad, as a student you should still apply the advice in this guidance wherever possible.

In addition to the above, if you get the opportunity to type in the notes always sign them clearly, stating your name and PHYSICIAN ASSOCIATE STUDENT and then whichever doctor, PA or healthcare professional has reviewed the patient. If you have not finished writing the notes and are called away to do something else, it is always good to write *notes unfinished* or similar.

Top tips

- Be honest – if someone asks you a question that you do not know the answer to, that's OK. You are a student, and they are expecting to teach you. If a patient asks you a question that you are not sure about, be honest and say that you will ask a senior.
- Don't pretend to be a medical student. You are a PA student and that is something to be proud of!

Potential areas for concern around professionalism

- Persistent inappropriate attitude or behaviour
- Failing to demonstrate good medical practice
- Drug or alcohol misuse
- Cheating or plagiarising
- Dishonesty or fraud, including dishonesty outside the professional role
- Aggressive, violent or threatening behaviour
- Any caution or conviction

Source: *Achieving Good Medical Practice* (GMC, 2016).

> Breaking confidentiality is also a cause for concern.

PA students will be able to get involved with much of the daily work of clinical practice whilst on placement. There will, however, be limitations as you are a student. It is important to know what you can do, and you should clarify this at your introductory meeting or induction sessions, as it may vary between practices or Trusts. For example, are you allowed (as a student) to:

- write in the notes?
- request blood tests?
- obtain blood cultures?
- print out blood forms?

In the Notes space below, jot down ideas of other tasks that you can find out whether you can do.

You should make sure that a qualified clinician reviews your patients.

 Notes

18.1 Medications prescription, supply and administration

As a PA student you are not permitted to prescribe, dispense, administer or to sign for administration of medications given to patients. For completion of your DOPS you are permitted to give I/M and S/C injections only under direct supervision of a qualified healthcare professional.

 Notes

19   Behaviour outside of university

As a PA student you need to behave professionally outside of work and university. This means you should avoid doing things that will undermine the trust patients have in PAs and the public has in the medical profession. For example, you should not make discriminatory comments about individuals or groups of people in public or on social media. Your university may take action if you do something unprofessional, such as get a caution for drunken behaviour, even if it happened outside of the university or over the summer holidays. This means you should take responsibility for your actions and be aware that they may have a wider impact on how your university views your professionalism.

Notes

Patients need to know that you are a student so they can make an informed decision about whether they want you to be involved in their care. Once they know you are a student, you can ask if they are happy for you to talk with them about their health or carry out a procedure. Remember:

- If you have any concerns about whether a patient has given consent to you being involved in their care or undertaking any type of procedure, talk to your supervisor about your concerns.
- You should be aware that sometimes patients might not have the capacity to give consent.
- You should not carry out any procedure on a patient without their consent for that specific procedure.
- You must respect the decision of patients who do not want you to be involved in their care.
- Don't forget to offer patients a chaperone. A chaperone must be present for intimate examinations.

 Top tip

- Don't be offended if a patient does not want to see you before seeing a qualified practitioner. It is nothing personal. You will get other opportunities; be patient.

Notes

How does confidentiality apply to my placements?

It is normal to want to talk about things you have seen on clinical placements with colleagues or friends. You will see unusual medical conditions and may be put in situations where patients experience adverse outcomes. You must **never** disclose patient-identifiable information without a patient's consent. If you are not sure what to share or if you are asked to provide information for an inquiry or logbook, you should ask for advice before you disclose any information.

Ensure any patient information you are given at placement – e.g. handover sheets – is put into confidential waste bins before you leave the site.

You should also make sure you never discuss patients in a public place or on social media. Even if you do not mention a patient by name, there is a chance that someone nearby (or online if you are on social media) might know whom you are talking about. If you do want to talk to a colleague, friend or supervisor about what you have seen on a placement, you should only do that in a private place and maintain patient anonymity. You should never mention the patient by name, except to a clinician directly involved in their care. For more information, see the GMC's guidance for registered doctors: *Good medical practice*, *Confidentiality* and *Doctors' use of social media*. You can find these at www.gmc-uk.org/guidance.

When writing your thoughts and statements in this book you must remember to preserve patient confidentiality and to only enter information which does not identify patients, staff or the organisation you are working in.

Guidance on using social media

Do:

- Check your privacy settings on any platforms that you use, so you know who can see things that you are posting. Remember that social media sites cannot guarantee confidentiality, whatever privacy settings you use.
- Maintain boundaries by not engaging with patients or others about a patient's care through your personal social media profiles or platforms. If someone contacts you directly, do not respond but escalate it to your placement team.
- Remember that once information is published on social media sites you may not be able to control how it is used by others. Even when a post is deleted, it can be difficult to ensure that it is completely removed from the internet or the site it was originally posted on.
- Use social media to express your views, but do not behave in a derogatory manner to other users and do not post discriminatory content. Think carefully about how others, particularly patients both present and future, might perceive your content.

Don't:

- Share information about patients or post information that could identify a patient.
- Add any information which can identify the Trust or practice that you are on placement with.
- Misrepresent your skills or level of training to others.
- Post complaints about your placement providers, university, teachers or trainers.

The patient should always be at the centre of all that we do and any decisions that are made about them or their care. Whilst this may seem obvious and an inherent part of what we should do as healthcare professionals, on some occasions it does not happen. Take time to talk to your patients and include them in all decisions about their care.

Top tip

- Treat patients as you would like your family members or yourself to be treated.

Notes

Settling there

24 | First day – what to expect

As stated in *Section 15*, you will have received first day reporting instructions in advance of starting your placement or have been given contact details for your supervisor, for you to make contact and find out where and when you should start your placement. Make sure that you arrive in plenty of time and that you know where you must get to. It is advisable to try to arrive 15 minutes before your expected reporting time, as sometimes you may have to present to a reception area and sign in before being able to arrive at the location.

You should be given an induction – this may be as part of a scheduled induction in advance of your placement, or it may be a personalised induction to your clinical area on your first morning. During your first day, make sure you familiarise yourself with any emergency procedures such as fire escape routes, emergency call numbers and equipment. If you have any queries or concerns, make sure you raise them with an appropriate member of staff such as a ward manager, practice manager or your supervisor.

You may be issued with an ID card for the organisation; this should clearly identify you as a Physician Associate student. You should also make sure that you wear any university ID badges that you may have been issued for identification.

 Notes

Top tips – Preparation

- Be confident when arriving in the clinical area. Make sure that you know where you are meant to be and who you are meeting. Introduce yourself clearly and professionally.
- Find out where you might be able to keep your belongings. If you are unable to determine this in advance, consider taking the 'bare minimum' on your first day until you understand the setting a little better.
- Consider making yourself a packed lunch for the first day, as you may not have access to a food outlet. It might be best to have food that does not require refrigeration or microwave cooking, until you know if you will have access to these facilities.

 Notes

All PA students should be allocated an overall medical placement supervisor, regardless of which clinical setting they are placed in. This is the person who is responsible for your time at the placement site. You may or may not work with your supervisor all the time, and it is likely that you will be supervised or supported by other members of the medical / multidisciplinary team throughout your placement; this will vary between placement type and settings.

Ultimately, as PAs practise medicine, the supervision, support and oversight of the student experience is primarily expected from the medical team. However, there may be times – for example while carrying out a procedure – when the best and most competent person to supervise and support you may be from another healthcare professional group. You should discuss during the first week of the placement how your supervision will work.

If you require sign-off for placement, again you should discuss with your supervisor how this will be done and who will do it. If your supervisor will be completing your sign-off but you have not worked with them for any significant period, ask if they will be seeking feedback from those you have been working with. This will help reassure you that this is a fair process and a truer reflection of your capabilities.

All patients that you see on placement must be reviewed by a medically qualified practitioner.

Top tips – Supervision

- Tag along with the nurses and trainee doctors for procedural skills where you can.
- Consider how you address qualified colleagues when you are on placement; you may be invited to use first names, but this should not be done in front of patients.
- Try to get your DOPS or other assessments signed off where opportunities arise.

 Notes

26 | Timetable

Many placements will issue students with a timetable, to plan their time alongside other students in the setting. If you have been timetabled to be in a specific clinic, then you are expected to be on time and prepared. Most schedules are flexible; however, if you are given one it is best to follow it. If at any point in the schedule you are not going to be where it states you should be, then you need to speak with your supervisor about this.

If there is no set schedule, then you can ask what a typical week is like and create a schedule from this. You can ask about ward rounds, clinics, teaching, and who the team or people are that you will be working with daily. As a student it is important to be visible and to discuss and communicate any changes. It will help solve problems later if the supervisor is querying where you have been during the placement.

For placements such as A&E, timings may be less rigid. Try to attend placement at various times of the day so that you can experience diverse types of patients and presentations. Ensure that this is agreed by your placement supervisor, that you have appropriate supervision and that your university programme is also aware.

 Top tip – Teaching

- Whilst you are on placement primarily to gain clinical experience, it's always good to ask if there is any teaching that would be suitable for you to attend. This is usually for staff employed there, although there may be some specifically for students. It is a good opportunity to show that you are using your initiative; it can also be very helpful in terms of keeping up to date with current guidelines.

You will need to stay in the clinical environment which has been allocated to you and not head into other departments. For example, if you are taking part in a paediatrics placement, you should remain based with the paediatrics team and not head over to acute medicine "because there's lots going on". This can be arranged but should be in exceptional circumstances only, and requires discussion and agreement of both your clinical supervisors and the university team. Similarly, you should not be spending huge amounts of time studying in the library, as this is not clinical placement (tempting for many students, particularly leading up to exams). Instead, focus on getting the hands-on practical experience with real patients which will support you in your path to becoming a safe and competent clinician.

If you are not going to be able to attend an activity which has been timetabled for you, ensure that you inform the team. Not doing so is unprofessional and sends a poor message.

 Challenge yourself – Timetabling

- Find out what time your day should start – for example ward rounds on surgical and medical wards may often differ, clinic times in general practice may vary across the week, or there may be a handover between the night and day team in a particular office.
- Speak to PAs or doctors in your clinical area about pre-reading for specialist clinics, meetings (such as X-ray meeting, MDTs) or other clinical events in your timetable, to make sure that you are appropriately prepared.
- Ask your course if there is a student 'tips and tricks' document which might also have access to some useful hints to maximise your placement.

Take the time to introduce yourself to everyone you will be working with, tell them what your role is and what you need to achieve. You are a member of the team, and you will get much more out of the placement if people know who you are and what you are there to do.

Many PA students frequently get asked about their backgrounds and their career choice – this is still a relatively new career and people are genuinely curious about those who have chosen to embark on it. Feel free to be honest in your response, but be professional and consider that as a PA student you have an ambassadorial responsibility.

It is worth bearing in mind that you may be the first PA student on that placement or in the organisation that the medical, or wider healthcare team has worked with. It is useful to be able to talk a little about your course and what is happening in the world of PAs – for example, they may ask if you know about whether PAs will be able to prescribe in the future, as they try to understand more not only about you as a student but also about the wider professional picture. You could utilise the Faculty of Physician Associates website (fparcp.co.uk) to make sure that you are up to date with any significant changes in the profession, as well as the updates from the FPA via your course student representative.

 Notes

Challenge yourself – Introductions

- Practise saying who you are and what a PA is. Have some blurb ready, and make what you have to say your own rather than formulaic (also make sure it is correct!)
- Practise answering questions that you might be asked about what a PA is and what they do. Speak to your course team about this before you go on placement if you aren't sure how to respond.
- Know the resources available to help you point people in the right direction for further information.

 Notes

Communication and examination are key skills for a PA student to practise on placement in preparation for exams (OSCEs) but also for preparation as a qualified PA. Practising these skills will help you build confidence and competence. It is important to remember when examining or speaking to patients that these are real people and not manikins to practise on, and that staff are there to deliver essential care.

28.1 Communication with patients

Poor communication is a leading cause of adverse events in healthcare, so developing your communication skills as a Physician Associate student is vital. When speaking with patients you will have been taught and had opportunities to practise communication skills in your programme and most likely will have developed a range of communication tools to use in different situations. Examples of these might include:

- How to take a history from a patient (open and closed questions, summarising, following patient cues, signposting)
- Explaining a procedure, test results or an examination (checking patients' current knowledge and understanding, chunking and checking)
- Breaking bad news to a patient (warning shot, pauses, no false reassurance)
- Explaining how to take a medication and checking understanding (gathering brief information, clear instructions, safety-netting).

28.2 Communication with other healthcare professionals

Speaking to other healthcare professionals can be daunting to start with. Presenting back a patient takes time and skill. You will need to practise doing this. When speaking to other healthcare professionals about a patient who is unwell or whom you are concerned about, the SBARD (Situation, Background, Assessment, Recommendation, Decision) framework is a useful and recognised tool for relaying important information effectively and concisely.

Situation	Concise statement of the problem
Background	Pertinent and brief information related to the situation
Assessment	Analysis and considerations of options – what you found / think
Recommendation	Action requested / recommended – what you want
Decision	Action taken

28.3 Examination of patients

Before examining a patient, you must always seek their consent and offer a chaperone (as mentioned in *Section 20*). Always tell the patient what the examination will involve, to prepare them for what is to come. Remember to use clear language and no jargon and to give clear instructions as to what they need to do. Think about patient dignity in every examination and drape / cover patients appropriately. Use a structured approach to your examinations, such as 'Inspect, Palpate, Percuss and Auscultate' for most examinations (IPPA), and the principles of 'Look, Feel and Move' for musculoskeletal examinations. You may need to modify your examinations depending on the patient and the environment that you are in. Do not carry out any examinations or procedures that you have not been taught to do. Never cut corners and never make up an examination finding. It is good if you can get someone to observe you carry out your examination and provide you with constructive feedback. This may be another student, member of the team or your supervisor.

 Top tips – Communication and examination of patients

- What worked well?
- What did not work well?
- What will you do next time?

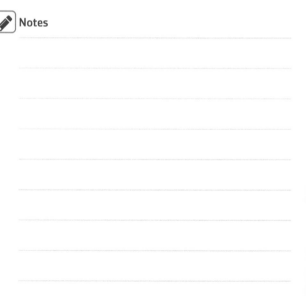

Notes

Being there

Being a student as part of a healthcare team is a privilege and comes with several responsibilities. You are there to learn, to contribute to the clinical care of patients under supervision, to experience life in the clinical setting, and to get a broader understanding of what it is to be part of the healthcare team. You will be able to witness some truly life-changing events for patients, and to work closely with the team providing that care. You will see people being born, people dying, and anything in between. As a PA student, or indeed anyone in healthcare, you are in the privileged position of seeing patients at their most vulnerable and having them trust you to act appropriately. You will witness emotional highs and lows; acute and longer-term problems; and the chance to truly comprehend the value and benefits of providing excellent patient care to all. It is important to remember that patients who are unwell or staff who are stressed do not always behave as they would when they are well or not stressed. This is not a reason to accept abuse, but just to help keep things in perspective.

As a student, it is important to understand that learning on placement is your priority and that this needs to be balanced against patient experience and choice, and especially patient safety. Your supervisors, and the wider supporting team, will be able to help you to meet this balance, for example by sourcing or recommending suitable patients for you to speak with to practise your history-taking skills. Some patients may not wish to be assessed or treated by a student, and this is their right – if you find yourself in this situation then be polite and ensure that the team you are working with are aware of this.

It is important to make sure that tasks which you are unable to complete are handed over to the medical team working with you on that day. For example, if you were asked by the FY1 to take some blood tests, but you were unable to get the sample, the team must know; not to do so would cause unnecessary delays and potentially harm to the patient.

Top tips for PA students from other healthcare professions

- If you have entered the PA profession from a different profession, it is crucial to remember that you are on placement as a PA student. You may have additional skills and experiences, but it is key to ensure that you do not carry out tasks outside of your scope of practice.
- Similarly, it is important to make sure that you try to resist the 'comfort' in the familiarity of your old role.

Notes

To get the very most out of your placements, you should try to have as much patient contact as possible. You should liaise with the clinical team to ensure that you understand all the opportunities available; for example, if the midwife runs a clinic in the GP practice on a Thursday morning, speak to the practice manager or GP supervisor to see if you might be able to join them to see a few patients.

Be prepared to take notes to aid your learning, but do not rely on having lots of free time to be able to read up about them. As a PA student, you are enrolled on a busy, intensive course with little downtime. Try to get into the habit of reading as you go, and learn about a new condition, test or procedure that you encountered every day. If you have questions following a ward round or after your GP has reviewed a patient, then you should ask the people you are working with. If they are busy, write these questions down and ask them at a later point when there may be more time, or ask another member of the team where appropriate.

Consider the environment and 'read the room' – the assessment of a rapidly deteriorating patient or a crash call are not appropriate times to be asking questions about the evidence base behind clinical choices; the clinicians will be focused on their job and your questions will be a hindrance. Instead, ask at the end if they could spare you a moment at a convenient time to debrief on what you witnessed, to ensure you understood what was happening.

Follow the progress of your patients – if you see a patient in the Emergency Department or Medical Assessment Unit, follow up with that patient in a couple of days – what has happened since their admission, how are they getting on? Many patients enjoy seeing students whom they encountered on admission and updating them about their progress. It is also a fantastic way to see if the management plans put in place have worked or if they have changed. This helps with confidence in your clinical decision making and management plans for patients. In primary care, see if the patients are booked for a further consultation and make a point of saying hello when possible or keeping a note of these patients and checking out what happened to them. Have they reattended? Did the treatment work? If they were referred, what was the outcome of the referral?

Remember, some wards will have policies about giving patients rest periods, so you may find that you have to come back later if they are about to have a meal or have visitors. The ward managers or nurse-in-charge will usually be able to inform you of these.

On GP and secondary care placements you can also ask for interesting cases related to systems / patient presentations you are covering at university. This can help consolidate your knowledge, give you an opportunity to practise your history taking and physical examination skills and to review the patient journey.

 Notes

Top tips – Seizing opportunities

- Always think ahead before your supervising PA or doctor tells you the plan for each patient. What investigations would you want to do? What treatments do you think are appropriate? What teams need to get involved? Do they need follow-up?
- Ask relevant questions – it helps your learning and shows that you are taking an interest in what's happening.
- Practise summarising to your supervisor as much as you can. If a consultant has time to hear your summary, give it a go.
- Get involved, even if it scares you – whether that's putting in a cannula, taking a history, referring a patient over the phone, or something else, now is the time to practise things you don't feel confident with.
- If you get the opportunity to present in a grand round or to the team, take it. You may feel terrified, but you'll learn a lot from it, and can gain valuable feedback for future presentations.

Notes

Making your own opportunities

A placement is usually successful because the student gets involved in many different aspects of their clinical area. During your placement, make sure that you take the initiative, and speak to the junior medical team, nurses, Allied Health Professionals (AHPs), nurse practitioners, administrators, reception staff and other staff members about their roles in the clinical environment and how they contribute to patient care.

If you have some space in your timetable, and do not have any specific tasks given to you, ask the team if you can be of any help (they may not know what skills you have, and so won't ask you to do jobs unless you offer – remember you may be one of the first PA students that they have worked with). Ask if you can shadow or tag along with someone.

Often you may find that you are told that there is nothing "interesting to do"; however, there is always plenty to do (whether "interesting" or not) – any experience is useful. If you're present on the morning ward round, take a note of patients that you could later examine or take a history from and ask them for their consent and whether there is a suitable time for you to come and do this in the afternoon; many patients appreciate the advance warning that you would be keen to come back to chat to them (providing the team haven't already got jobs for you to do). Ward round can be a good time to find opportunities for yourself later in the day, e.g. bloods, changing cannulas, finding good patients to take a history or examine.

Challenge yourself – Patient history

- Take a history from a patient who has already been admitted to hospital. Don't read their notes before you start. Come up with your own diagnosis and differential diagnosis, treatment and management plan. Once you have completed this, go and read the patient notes to see how much of it matches what is written in the admission notes.
- If you've got a good match, well done! Reflect on what the key points were from the history that pointed you to that particular diagnosis.
- Don't worry if you've not got it quite right, instead reflect on what you may have missed from the history, or diagnoses that you did not consider.

Other valuable learning opportunities which will not be timetabled may include (but are not limited to):

- Talking to admitted patients about their presenting complaints (practising your history-taking skills) and how their condition has changed with treatment
- Understanding management plans by reading the patient records, drug charts and hospital protocols
- Assessing a patient with physiotherapists, occupational therapists or other AHPs
- Shadowing a nurse on a medication round and becoming familiar with medications being used in a particular area
- Sitting in with a practice nurse running a chronic disease clinic, and considering the value of patient education to support the management of their chronic condition
- Performing a medication review with a ward-based or practice-based pharmacist
- Accompanying a patient for imaging or other investigation or procedure
- Setting up a 'team' with some other students and presenting cases to each other along with some key learning points

- Participating in audits or other projects happening in the Trust or practice; this is useful for your CV, so keep a note (appropriately anonymised) of the project and your involvement
- Presenting cases at ward or Trust meetings to the medical team or to other students
- Reviewing patient notes or following up on patients that you have seen in the primary or secondary care environment to see the outcomes based on decisions made or the management plan.

The more you put into these experiences, the more you get out of them. This is your opportunity to show that PAs can become a valuable part of the team, as well as helping you to become a safe and competent medical healthcare practitioner.

1 Top tips from PA students on placements

- Ask if there is anything you can help with. The more you offer, the more people will trust you and invite you to help them.
- Bring some revision with you (e.g. DEARSIM (Definition, Epidemiology, Aetiology, Risk factors, Signs/symptoms, Investigations, Management) or the *Top 100 Drugs* book) or coursework so that you can maximise your time at placement if there is downtime between clinics, for example, or to read when you are travelling.
- Asking for help is a good thing. Staff are so happy to help and are used to working as a team. It's much more important that the patient gets what they need.
- Try to be as sociable as possible. Have lunch in communal areas or if possible, with the team. Try not to always be on your phone or your laptop.
- Always bear in mind upcoming assignments so you can pick a good patient to write about. Keeping a record or a log can help with this.

Your course should ensure that you have a clear understanding of assessments and documentation required during each placement. This may include (but is not limited to):

- Timesheets/attendance sheets – filled in and signed off daily/weekly
- Logging patients (either in a portfolio or on an online system)
- Case-based discussions
- Multi Source Feedback (team assessment of behaviours)
- Clinical skills passports
- Mini-CEX or equivalent
- And any number of other assessments required.

Before you start your clinical placements, most programmes will offer a supporting taught session to ensure that you understand the requirements. Do not hesitate to contact the placement lead or appropriate member of the PA course team if you have any questions or concerns about your assessments whilst on placement.

Most programmes will require a 'sign-off' from the supervisor at the end of the placement, so ensure that you factor in the time for this and be prepared to initiate the conversation to book some time for this assessment.

 Notes

What to do if things go wrong

Given the proportion of time that you will spend on placement during the PA course, the likelihood is that you will experience something going wrong at some point. These are usually minor things, with no significant consequences, but it is important to remember that it is essential to stay calm and professional throughout, regardless of the size of the issue or concern.

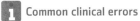 Common clinical errors

- Misidentification of patients
- Mislabelling bottles
- Drug errors
- Spillages and contamination events
- Miscommunication
- Errors by omission
- Needlestick injuries

> Such events, whilst not uncommon, must be reported and you will need to follow hospital policy. Do not feel embarrassed, and always seek help.

If you experience any problems that may prevent the progress or satisfactory completion of the placement, you should speak to the PA academic team on your course as soon as you are able. Forewarned is certainly forearmed in such situations, and it is advisable to let the team know of any potential issues before they become a problem. You should, as part of the placement preparation, be given a contact to report any concerns or issues to; this might be the clinical placement lead on the teaching team, the administrative team, or both.

You may wish to engage with the Student Services team (or equivalent) where required, particularly if you are considering if you might need to take a step back or have some prolonged absence for any reason.

You should also speak to the team at the university if you have concerns or complaints about specific matters of concern (whistleblowing) whilst on placement. Many universities have concern forms which can be completed to highlight any issues a student may wish to raise. Alternatively you may wish to email the placement lead directly to initiate further discussion. Ensure that you seek support from the university if you are involved in or witness a situation which causes you distress.

Some of our greatest learning happens when things do not go to plan and whilst at the time it may be challenging, it is good when the situation resolves to try to objectively reflect on what happened. It will enable you to recognise and prevent the situation arising again and or aid you to manage it in a more effective way in the future.

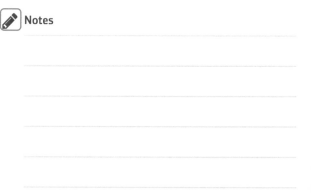 **Notes**

Regular meetings with supervisor / team

It is important that you have regular meetings with your supervisor, or appointed alternative member of staff, throughout your placement. The number of meetings will vary depending on the length of placement but as a minimum, it is recommended that you meet with your supervisor within the first couple of days, at some point in the middle of the placement and then at the end for sign-off. Some students may have extended placements of several months in the same place, in which case it would be appropriate for multiple 'catch-ups' during that middle period. Other placements may only be 2 or 3 weeks long.

The purpose of these meetings is to check on how you are getting on, what you have achieved thus far or what you need to achieve moving forward, how you will do that, and that you are on track to meet placement objectives. Be prepared for these meetings, bring any paperwork that may require review or sign-off and anything else that you wish to discuss. It is necessary that you understand what you are trying to get out of the meetings and for it to be a useful endeavour for all concerned. By understanding the aims, you are able to prepare for the meetings appropriately, as well as being able to drive the conversation where required.

 Notes

Meeting type	Suggested timeframe
Initial meeting	Within first 2 or 3 days of placement
Intermediate catch-ups	At regular intervals (every other week as a minimum) on longer placement; may only meet once, or not be required on some shorter placements
Final meeting	Within final 2 or 3 days of placement

Aim of meeting	Suggested preparation
To understand the scope of the placement – ensuring that you have a plan to meet the required learning outcomes as well as address any further interests in the specialty To understand the expectations of your supervisor, potential to get a view on whether placement will be timetabled or student-driven. If the latter, ensure you understand where to get more information, e.g. secretary, other colleagues within the team	Review the learning outcomes for the placement Reflect on your own development – is there any learning that you particularly want to focus on?
As suggested in the name – touch base to discuss any new questions or concerns; showcase progress and learning; discuss how to achieve remaining outcomes	Review learning outcomes and performance against those established at first meeting Be able to discuss what you have done with your time, what has been useful (or not) / interesting / surprising, and what you need help with Be prepared to discuss a case that you have seen and learnt from whilst on current placement
To review whether learning objectives have been met and complete any required placement documentation / assessments To evaluate performance and receive feedback on how to get the most out of future placements (feed forward) Final placement sign-offs, e.g. time / attendance sheets / DOPS / competency assessments	Review learning outcomes and performance against those established at first meeting Be able to discuss what you have done with your time, what has been useful (or not)/interesting/surprising Be prepared to discuss a case that you have seen and learnt from whilst on current placement

It is vitally important that you take the time to look after yourself whilst on placement. It is incredibly easy to get caught up in a busy clinical day, seeing lots of patients and taking advantage of every opportunity, then coming home and reading up on all the new things that you have seen, without giving a thought to any downtime or time to relax. Or worse still, feeling guilty about taking some time to relax and recuperate.

Top tips – Self-care

- Don't beat yourself up if you do not have time to revise every day. Remember, if you are getting involved, you can learn something with every patient! You are actively revising during your shifts.
- Talk to your peers if you feel comfortable doing so. They are likely to be feeling the same and know how intense the course can be. If you struggle to feel motivated to revise, try meeting up in a group and then reward yourselves with downtime together afterwards.

 Notes

Eating right, getting enough sleep and exercising regularly are all things that we know can help to support better mental health, alongside making time for your hobbies and interests. You need to ensure that you have time to do things that interest you – go to the gym, go for a walk, see friends and family, watch a movie... whatever floats your boat, that ensures that you have some time for your brain to switch off and think about something unrelated. The most important thing is to ensure that you have the balance right – too much time studying can lead to you being tired and unable to contribute to your highest standard, but not enough studying clearly isn't the answer either. Time management is key here – set yourself clear times when you will study, and when you will have some time off to enjoy yourself. Then make sure that you stick to those – make sure friends, housemates or family are aware too so they can support you in your schedule, and you'll be able to go to placement prepared but also well rested and ready to perform.

You may see things on placement that may have a profound effect on you; a trauma, an angry patient, a difficult consultation or the death of a patient whom you have spent time with. Do not underestimate the impact that these situations may have. It is important that you speak with your team or supervisor to debrief where possible. If this is not possible speak to your course team or seek support from the university student support services. It is important to speak about these things, to reflect on the impact that they have had and identify any learning from them.

Burnout is increasingly apparent across healthcare professionals and healthcare students, so it is absolutely key to your development that you can take some time away from the rigours of clinical medicine. The RCP has an online resource focused on Mental Health and Wellbeing, with tools to help you to identify issues and recognise possible triggers, and strategies to help you to be able to open the conversation and seek support in getting help. There are also several apps available, such as Headspace, SilverCloud, Unmind, Sleepio, which have been shown to help to take some time to look after yourselves.

Remember that you also have access to the wealth of student wellbeing and support resources via your university. If you are not coping with your placements, or need to discuss your situation with someone, you should engage with your personal tutor, university teams, student support services or other services based at the university. If you are not sure who to contact, speak to your course or placement lead to raise a concern (this can be done without giving details if preferred); they can then signpost accordingly.

Notes

Moving on

You may be asked to formally complete a portfolio of patients that you see during your clinical placements, or log the details in some other way. Regardless of whether you will be asked to formally submit a portfolio or not, it is important for your learning that you take some time to reflect on some of your clinical encounters to ensure that you are not only developing your clinical knowledge but also your experiences and understanding as a medical healthcare student.

Reflective practice is often required as part of Continuing Professional Development (CPD) evidence – this is currently true as part of the RCP CPD Diary for PAs (used by FPA members) – and is an essential skill for you to develop as a PA and as part of the healthcare workforce of the future.

There are many different methods for reflection. There is no *right way* to reflect, although you may find that your PA course offers you a suggested model (Gibbs' and Johns' models are frequently used). Sometimes, you may just think through a case on your own, and do some further reading about one of the issues arising from it. At other times, it may be more appropriate to discuss as a larger group of students, or with your supervisor to work through some of the intricacies. The GMC offers guidance for medical students around developing as a reflective practitioner, including tools to help you understand what works for you, considering when to reflect and with whom, as well as some examples of good practice. Review the guidance at bit.ly/GMC-36

> To make it easy for you to access them, we have shortened some web links to this format – simply type these into any web browser and you'll go to the right page! Do note that they are case sensitive.

Preparation for the next placement

For many PA students, you will be required to go immediately from one placement to the next, without any clear time for reflection and processing before you're 'new' again in a different setting, having to repeat the cycle. This can be exhausting, so please do ensure that you are prepared, and make sure you read *Section 35* about self-care.

Your next placement may be in the same place – for example, a different ward or specialty within the same hospital – but alternatively may be somewhere completely different. You need to ensure that you can prepare yourself – find out reporting instructions, understand where you need to go (including a 'dry run' if somewhere new), consider if you need to do any pre-reading (you can also ask this question in the email to your supervisor – it shows you are engaged and proactive from the start!), at the same time as continuing to work to a high standard on your current placement. This can be tricky, and requires some balance, but with some foresight and planning, it is doable. It is important to consider your ambassadorial role as a PA student, and not lower your standards or take time off the wards to investigate your next placement, unless by prior arrangement and in discussion with your PA course.

 Notes

Top tips – Planning future placements

- Good relationships with fellow students will be key here. Keep in contact with each other and learn from each other's experiences – this will make a lot of the preparation much easier.
- Try to maintain your studies throughout, so you are not going into your next placement with a feeling that you're behind in your reading.
- If possible, try to do some longer-term preparation before your placements start – keep a folder with headings such as 'pre-reading topics' and 'key points from other students', as well as consolidating your learning into some short summaries of key medical topics. You can then pull out the relevant page before each particular placement starts and feel more confident.

 Notes

Throughout your placements, you will have seen and done many things as well as gained valuable knowledge and skills. These will help you grow and develop and prepare you for professional practice as a qualified PA. We would strongly recommend that you keep a record of your experiences, knowledge and skills, as this will help you to develop good habits and begin your professional portfolio. You can use your professional portfolio to demonstrate your achievements to employers and for review and appraisal purposes. Keeping a record of what you have been learning will also enable you to identify gaps that you can then address in future placements and in self-directed learning and revision.

 Challenge yourself – Reflection

- Consider the patients that you have seen on a particular placement. Identify gaps in your clinical experience and knowledge from your placement, as well as reviewing outstanding assessments or sign-offs.
- Use these to formulate a plan for moving onward:
  - Can these be addressed in future placements?
  - What do you need to focus on and see next time?
  - Can you do some further reading about the topics?

 Notes

Feedback is a two-way street, working in both directions. As part of your placement, you should have an end of placement review with your clinical supervisor, where you should receive feedback about your performance on the placement, as well as having the opportunity to ask any questions or raise any discussion points that you may have. Make sure that this meeting is scheduled when you start the placement and check the week before that your clinical supervisor is still available to meet. If they are no longer available check with them to see who else might be able and appropriate to sign you off.

> If, as part of your placement, you haven't spent much time with your clinical supervisor, for example due to on-call rotas or annual leave, then please speak to those whom you have spent time with and ask them to drop a note to your clinical supervisor about you – it will be helpful for both of you to get some more meaningful feedback.

You may have paperwork which needs to be completed at this stage, for example Placement Assessment Documents or other review forms. Many PA programmes now have these available online. It is useful to ensure that you have both an electronic version and a paper version handy, just in case your supervisor has not received a copy or in case of other issue, to allow it to be completed as part of your review session. It is possible to get such documents filled in after the event, but much more challenging.

You should also be asked to complete a placement evaluation giving your perspective of the placement. This may be part of the assessment document or may be a separate process. Many universities will collate these evaluations, and then provide the placement sites with their feedback, which has been anonymised. Please be honest about your experience, even if it is a less than positive experience. Your PA course will consider your feedback when allocating future placements, so need a clear idea about how it works on a day-to-day basis and if it is a successful placement. If you did encounter problems, avoid just venting – successful feedback involves constructive criticism, so make sure that you give your perspective on what would make it better. If you had a positive experience, ensure that you report that on your feedback form, and particularly mention any members of staff who made your placement particularly successful / enjoyable, as they will then be able to record this as part of their own records towards their portfolios or appraisals.

 Challenge yourself – Share your successes

Make time to send an email to your placement lead, or get involved in a discussion with other students at an academic in-day and share your successes! This is useful for the team to understand what the students are doing, as well as having an opportunity to celebrate your hard work with you and the other students.

 Top tip – Feedback

Welcome any feedback. Don't be defensive if you receive negative feedback – it is all constructive and staff all want the best for your learning experience!

✎ Notes

Resources

- PC – Presenting Complaint
- HPC – History of Presenting Complaint
- PMH – Past Medical History – (include pertinent positives, pertinent negatives and red flags)
- Medications – (include dose, frequency, when commenced, route of administration, OTC, recreational and concordance)
- Allergies – (include what the reaction is)
- Family History – (including anything particularly related to the HPC)
- Social History – (including anything particularly related to the HPC)
- RoS – Review of Systems
- Physical Examination – appropriate to the HPC
- Impression/Diagnosis (Dx) / Differential Dx
- Investigations (Ix)
- Management (Mx)

Can use SOCRATES for a history of pain (Site; Onset; Character; Radiation; Associated symptoms; Time; Exacerbating/relieving factors; Severity)

VINDICATE, VITAMIN C DEFK, or ACTIVEE MINDS as mnemonics for aetiologies for differential diagnosis:

- Vascular; Infections/Inflammatory; Neoplastic; Degenerative/Drug; Iatrogenic/Intoxication; Congenital; Autoimmune/Allergy; Traumatic; Endocrine/Environment; Metabolic/Mechanical; Behavioural; Social; Karyotype; Functional

Patients <u>must always</u> be reviewed by someone medically qualified.

If writing in patient notes, always clearly sign name and state designation – PA Student.

Presenting a patient

This is a skill to learn – practice is key!

- Patient details – name, DOB/age, ethnicity, gender born and where appropriate they/them if non-binary
- PC – can include if patient has any long-term chronic conditions or highlight any pertinent information – e.g. Mrs Brown has presented with chest pain on a background of unstable angina and type 2 diabetes mellitus
- HPC – patient story – succinct with pertinent positives and negatives of the HPC
- Medications and Allergies
- Family and Social History – pertinent/relevant details
- RoS any additional information not directly relevant to the HPC but a problem for the patient
- Physical examination findings
- Investigations requested and results or investigations that will be requested
- Management of the patient so far and the proposed plan

 Notes

Common examinations, tests, investigations, and scoring / risk assessment tools, by system

SYSTEM	Examinations	Investigations
Cardiovascular (CVS)	CVS exam Peripheral vascular exam	Brain natriuretic peptide (BNP) Troponin Creatine kinase Cholesterol & lipid profile HbA1c Chest X-ray Ultrasound scan (USS) (triple AAA)
Respiratory	Respiratory examination	Chest X-ray ABG Computed tomography pulmonary angiography (CTPA) Pulse oximetry Fractional exhaled nitric oxide (FeNO) Mantoux test

cedures	Assessment / scoring tools	What they assess
+/− erect and supine +/− t and left arm)	CHA_2DS_2-VASc	Risk of stroke
	HAS-BLED	Risk of major bleeding in patients requiring anticoagulation for AF
rcise stress test	QRISK3	Likelihood of developing CVD/stroke
48-hour tape (Holter itoring)	Body mass index (BMI)	If someone is over-/underweight
onary angiogram	Framingham Risk Score	Estimates 10-year risk of heart attack
cardiocentesis		
	New York Heart Association (NYHA)	Stratifies severity of heart failure by symptoms
	PACK years	Calculates number of pack years in patients with smoking history
k flow	CURB65 (creatine; urea; respiratory rate; blood pressure; age >65)	Secondary care – severity of pneumonia and treatment
ometry		
tum sample	CRB65 – as above without urea	Primary care (as above)
nchoscopy		
racentesis	Wells criteria	Risk of PE/DVT
ral tap	PERC rule	Rule out criteria for PE
	MRC dyspnoea scale	Breathlessness severity scoring system
	Epworth Sleepiness Score	Used in the assessment of suspected obstructive sleep apnoea

SYSTEM	Examinations	Investigations
Gastrointestinal (GI)	GI examination Rectal examination	Abdo X-ray USS *Helicobacter pylori* (*H. pylori*) CLO-test or rapid urease test Stool culture micro-organisms and sensitivity (MC&S) Sigmoidoscopy Barium enema Barium swallow
Neurological	Cranial nerves Peripheral nerves	Electroencephalogram (EEG) Electromyography (EMG) CT head MRI brain PET scan Vit B12
Endocrine	Thyroid exam Diabetic foot exam	Thyroid function tests (TFT) Free T3/T4 HbA1c ACTH Aldosterone Hormones (FSH, LH, testosterone, oestrogen) Cortisol Prolactin Growth hormone Fine needle aspiration (FNA) USS CT MRI PET scan
Musculoskeletal	Neck and spine Shoulder Hand Hip Knee Foot and ankle	Inflammatory markers CRP ESR Rheumatoid factor X-ray USS DEXA bone scan

cedures	Assessment / scoring tools	What they assess
ophagogastroduodenoscopy D)	Rockall Score	Risk of rebleeding in those with an upper GI bleed
studies	Glasgow–Blatchford score	Assess need for admission in those with UGIB
onoscopy	Bristol Stool Chart	
oscopic retrograde angiopancreatography P)	CAGE questionnaire	Assesses alcohol use
	ROME diagnostic criteria	Criteria for diagnosis of IBS
tic tap	Child–Pugh	Scoring system to assess the severity of liver cirrhosis
	Gleason score	Indicates prognosis in prostate cancer
bar puncture	Glasgow Coma Scale (GCS)	
nal tap	Alert, new Confusion, responds to Voice, responds to Pain, Unresponsive (ACVPU)	Coma severity
	ABCD₂	Risk of stroke after TIA
od glucose monitoring (BM)		
siotherapy	Ottawa ankle rule	Rule out significant foot, ankle and knee fractures and reduces the use of X-ray
t injections	Ottawa knee rule	
ge-guided procedures	QFracture (NICE preferred)	To calculate risk of fragility fractures
gery	FRAX	
	DAS28	Measure of disease activity in rheumatoid arthritis

SYSTEM	Examinations	Investigations
Mental health	Mental health history	Mental state exam (MSE) Mini mental state exam (MMSE)
Female health	Breast exam Pelvic exam	Beta-hCG hormones (FSH, LH, testosterone, oestrogen) Prolactin High vaginal swabs Smear test Speculum exam
Male health	Penis, testicular & prostate exam	PSA
Dermatology	Skin	
ENT	Ear	{ Weber Rinne Dix–Hallpike
	Nose	{ Nasal speculum Swabs
	Throat	{ Monospot (EBV) Swabs
Ophthalmology	Eye exam – relevant cranial nerves	
Paeds	Relevant to presentation	Relevant to presentation Non-accidental injury
Other		

cedures	Assessment / scoring tools	What they assess
nitive behavioural therapy (T)	Generalised anxiety disorder (GAD)	Levels of anxiety
nselling		
chotherapy		
	PHQ-9	Score for degree of depression severity
	Mini mental state exam (MMSE)	Level of cognitive function score out of 30
	Abbreviated mental test score	Quick screening tool for level of cognitive function – score out of 10
	4AT	Rapid clinical test for delirium
oscopy	Pregnancy date calculators	Dates the pregnancy and expected date of delivery
terectomy		
horectomy		
mectomy		
ge loop excision of the sformation zone (LLETZ)		
ctoscope	Prostate-specific antigen score (PSA)	
oscopy		
	ABCDE melanoma criteria	Assessment of warning signs for melanoma
y manoeuvre	CENTOR score	Management of strep pharyngitis
	FeverPAIN score	Predicts likelihood of strep throat
rescein eye dye		
noval of a foreign body		
er presentation	APGAR	Neonates' health 1–5 minutes after birth
	Safeguarding	
	SEPSIS 6	Identification and rapid treatment of sepsis
	NICE rapid referral 2-week wait guidelines	Identification and rapid treatment of cancer

Arterial blood gas interpretation

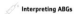

Interpreting ABGs

Step 1: Oxygenation

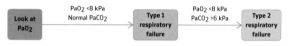

Step 2: Acid-base balance

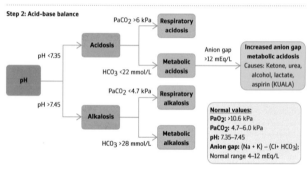

Reproduced with kind permission from gramproject.com.

Notes

Anaphylaxis guidelines

Anaphylaxis is a severe, potentially life-threatening allergic reaction.

- Patients having a reaction should be assessed and treated using the Airway, Breathing, Circulation, Disability, Exposure (ABCDE) approach.
- Most reactions occur quite quickly after exposure to an allergen. Signs of an anaphylactic reaction are:
  - patient is very anxious
  - airway swelling (tongue swelling, difficulty breathing and swallowing, feeling like their throat is closing)
  - shortness of breath
  - wheezing
  - patient is pale and/or clammy
  - tachycardia
  - hypotension
  - decrease/loss of consciousness
  - cardiac arrest.
- If necessary, depending on the patient's condition, carry out basic life support (see inside front cover).
- The patient's treatment plan will vary according to their location and the cause of the allergy.
- If an anaphylactic reaction occurred during medication administration/blood transfusion, make sure the IV is switched off.
- After an anaphylactic reaction patients should be referred to an allergy specialist.
- Intramuscular adrenaline is regarded as the treatment of choice (if a patient has a known allergy, to peanuts for example, they should carry their EpiPen at all times).
- Document in the notes what happened, the time and what action was taken.

There are occasions where you might be involved with people who have become acutely unwell. Acute physiological deterioration can occur for many reasons including infection, neurological insults, acute cardiac event, electrolyte disturbance, drug reaction, etc.

Physiological 'track and trigger' systems such as NEWS2 help healthcare professionals to identify a person who is deteriorating. Patient observations are used to create an aggregate score that then allows the team to make decisions regarding monitoring and management. Six simple physiological parameters form the basis of the screening system:

1. Respiration rate
2. Oxygen saturation
3. Systolic blood pressure
4. Pulse rate
5. Level of consciousness or new confusion
6. Temperature

 Notes

It is imperative that you seek help if you are the first person to identify an acutely ill patient. It is helpful to remember the ABCDE acronym to guide your assessment.

Airway	Check for airway patency – is the patient talking? Can you feel air flow? Are there abnormal breathing sounds or skin colour? If you have concerns about the patient's airway patency, shout for help and aim to secure the airway by using the head tilt, chin lift manoeuvre. Seek help for further airway support.
Breathing	Check respiratory rates, respiratory pattern and oxygen saturations (SpO_2). Respiratory rate changes are very sensitive indicators of physiological deterioration. Measure respiratory rate accurately – observe and count the patient's breaths over a full minute.
Circulation	Check blood pressure, heart rate and temperature. Palpate the radial pulse – is it regular and strong or irregular and weak? Do the extremities look blue or mottled? Do they feel cold to the touch?
Disability	Is the patient alert and oriented? Use the acronym ACVPU (Alert; new Confusion; responds to Voice; responds to Pain, Unresponsive). Are pupils an equal size and do they react to light?
Exposure	Head to toe check – are there rashes, signs of local infection, swelling, abdominal distension, wounds, drains? Remember to preserve dignity and comfort at all times.

Be sure to record your findings in the medical notes and have these countersigned by your clinical supervisor. Ensure that you communicate your findings and concerns to an appropriate member of the team.

There is a wide variety of applications available to support you on placement; speak to your PA programmes team who will be able to advise you about whether you can get access to the library online, with access to books such as *Oxford Handbooks* and other texts. There are many apps to guide knowledge in anatomy, keep knowledge up to date and offer patient resources. Some apps which previous students have found useful include:

- Induction app – directory of all the contact information for various departments
- British National Formulary (BNF)
- NICE CKS
- GP Notebook
- UpToDate
- Apps with OSCE and MCQ guidance, such as OSCE Stop, Geeky Medics, BMJ Best Practice
- MedCalc or other similar apps.

✎ **Notes**

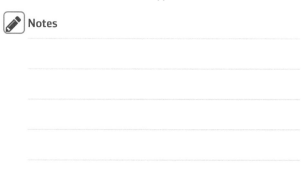

ACEPNow and Highland Ultrasound: highlandultrasound.com

Faculty of Physician Associates: fparcp.co.uk

GMC (2016) *Achieving Good Medical Practice.* Available at: bit.ly/GMC-47aa

GMC (2021) *Good Medical Practice: interim standards for physician associates and anaesthesia associates.* Available at: bit.ly/GMC-47bb

Gramproject: gramproject.com/diagram/arterial-blood-gas

How can you reflect? GMC online article. Available at: bit.ly/GMC-47c

Royal College of Physicians CPD Diary. Available at: bit.ly/RCP-47a

Royal College of Physicians Wellbeing Hub. Available at: bit.ly/RCP-47b

My Notes

My Notes

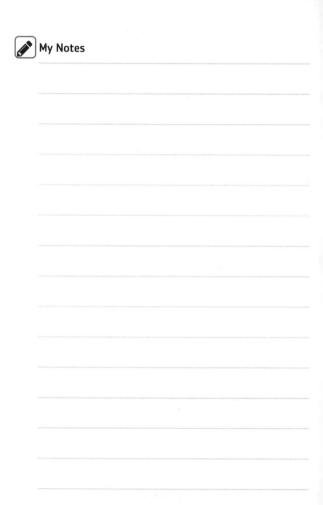

My Notes